PILATES REFORMER MASTERY:

Techniques for Total Body Transformation

SAM ABABIO

DEDICATION

To my family, whose unwavering support and love have been my foundation,

To my friends, who have inspired and encouraged me every step of the way,

And to all the dreamers and doers, who strive for success and never give up,

This book is dedicated to you.

May it be a guide and a source of inspiration on your journey to achieving your dreams.

With heartfelt gratitude.

TABLE OF CONTENT

Introduction

Overview of the Book

Welcome to **Pilates Reformer Mastery: Techniques for Total Body Transformation**. This book is designed to be your ultimate guide to mastering the Pilates Reformer, a powerful piece of equipment that can transform your body and elevate your fitness routine. Whether you're a beginner just starting your Pilates journey or an experienced practitioner looking to deepen your practice, this book provides comprehensive insights, detailed instructions, and practical tips to help you achieve your fitness goals.

Purpose and Goals of the Book

The primary purpose of this book is to demystify the Pilates Reformer and make its benefits accessible to everyone. The Pilates Reformer is often seen as an intimidating piece of equipment, but it is actually incredibly versatile and effective. This book aims to break down complex exercises into manageable steps, ensuring that readers of all levels can confidently use the Reformer to improve their strength, flexibility, balance, and overall fitness.

The goals of this book include:

1. **Education**: Provide a thorough understanding of the Pilates Reformer, including its history, benefits, and the core principles of Pilates that underpin all exercises.

2. **Instruction**: Offer clear, step-by-step instructions for a wide range of exercises, from basic to advanced, ensuring that readers can progress safely and effectively.
3. **Customization**: Help readers tailor their workouts to their specific needs and goals, whether they are looking to improve general fitness, rehabilitate an injury, or achieve specific performance targets.
4. **Inspiration**: Encourage readers to make Pilates a regular part of their fitness routine by highlighting the long-term benefits and providing motivational advice.

What Readers Will Achieve Through This Guide

By following this guide, readers will achieve a deeper understanding and mastery of the Pilates Reformer, leading to a range of physical and mental benefits:

1. **Improved Strength and Flexibility**: The Reformer offers resistance training that can enhance muscle tone and flexibility. Readers will learn exercises that target different muscle groups, promoting balanced strength throughout the body.
2. **Enhanced Core Stability**: Pilates is renowned for its focus on the core, and the Reformer takes this to the next level. Readers will discover techniques to strengthen their abdominal and back muscles, improving posture and reducing the risk of injury.

3. **Better Balance and Coordination**: The dynamic nature of Reformer exercises challenges balance and coordination, which can translate into improved performance in other physical activities and daily life.
4. **Increased Body Awareness**: Through precise movements and mindful practice, readers will develop greater body awareness, learning to move more efficiently and gracefully.
5. **Stress Reduction and Mental Clarity**: The mindful nature of Pilates promotes relaxation and mental clarity. Readers will learn to use breath and concentration to create a more focused and calm state of mind.
6. **Personalized Fitness Plans**: With guidance on creating customized workout routines, readers can design fitness plans that suit their individual needs, preferences, and goals.

This book is structured to provide a comprehensive journey through the world of Pilates Reformer. From understanding the fundamental principles and mastering basic techniques to advancing your practice and integrating Pilates into your lifestyle, each chapter builds on the last to ensure a complete and rewarding experience.

History and Benefits of Pilates

Origins and Evolution of Pilates

Pilates, a widely respected and practiced form of exercise, traces its origins back to the early 20th century. It was developed by Joseph Pilates, a German-born physical trainer with a passion for fitness and well-being. Joseph Pilates, influenced by his experiences in gymnastics, martial arts, yoga, and other physical training methods, created a unique system of exercises that emphasized core strength, flexibility, and overall body conditioning.

Early Life and Inspiration

Joseph Pilates was born in 1883 in Mönchengladbach, Germany. As a child, he suffered from various health issues, including asthma, rickets, and rheumatic fever. Determined to overcome these ailments, he embarked on a lifelong journey to improve his physical health. He studied anatomy, bodybuilding, wrestling, and Eastern disciplines like yoga and Zen meditation, integrating these diverse influences into his own exercise methodology.

Development of Contrology

During World War I, while interned in England as a German national, Joseph Pilates began developing his exercise system, which he initially called "Contrology." He worked with fellow internees, including those who were bedridden, using makeshift equipment like bed springs to create resistance exercises. This innovative approach laid the groundwork for the development of the Pilates Reformer and other specialized equipment.

Establishment of Pilates Studios

After the war, Joseph Pilates returned to Germany and continued refining his methods. In the 1920s, he immigrated to the United States, where he opened his first studio in New York City with his wife, Clara. Their studio attracted dancers, athletes, and actors, who appreciated the system's ability to enhance strength, flexibility, and overall body control. The Pilates method gained popularity in the performing arts community, with renowned dancers like Martha Graham and George Balanchine becoming advocates.

Evolution and Modernization

Over the decades, Pilates evolved as practitioners and instructors continued to develop and expand the original exercises. Today, Pilates is practiced worldwide, with a variety of styles and approaches. The introduction of modern equipment, such as the Pilates Reformer, Cadillac, and Wunda Chair, has further enhanced the versatility and effectiveness of the practice.

Key Benefits of Pilates for Physical and Mental Health

Pilates offers a multitude of benefits, encompassing physical, mental, and emotional well-being. Its holistic approach makes it a popular choice for individuals seeking a comprehensive fitness regimen.

Physical Benefits

1. **Core Strength and Stability**: Pilates is renowned for its emphasis on core strength. The

exercises target the deep abdominal muscles, obliques, and lower back, creating a strong and stable core that supports overall movement and posture.

2. **Flexibility and Range of Motion**: Pilates exercises promote flexibility and enhance the range of motion in joints. This is achieved through controlled, fluid movements that lengthen muscles and improve joint health.

3. **Balanced Muscle Development**: Unlike some forms of exercise that focus on specific muscle groups, Pilates ensures balanced development. It strengthens both the larger, primary muscles and the smaller, stabilizing muscles, promoting overall muscle balance and coordination.

4. **Improved Posture**: Pilates emphasizes alignment and posture, helping individuals develop awareness of their body's positioning. This leads to better posture, reduced strain on the spine, and a decreased risk of musculoskeletal issues.

5. **Injury Prevention and Rehabilitation**: The focus on controlled, precise movements makes Pilates an excellent choice for injury prevention and rehabilitation. It helps build strength and stability, reducing the risk of injuries and aiding in recovery from existing ones.

6. **Enhanced Athletic Performance**: Athletes often incorporate Pilates into their training routines to improve flexibility, core strength, and overall body awareness. This leads to enhanced performance in their respective sports.

Mental and Emotional Benefits

1. **Mind-Body Connection**: Pilates emphasizes the mind-body connection, requiring concentration and mindfulness during each exercise. This fosters a deeper awareness of one's body and movements, enhancing overall physical and mental coordination.
2. **Stress Reduction**: The controlled, rhythmic breathing techniques used in Pilates promote relaxation and reduce stress. This meditative aspect of Pilates can help alleviate anxiety and promote a sense of calm.
3. **Improved Focus and Concentration**: The precision and control required in Pilates exercises enhance mental focus and concentration. This can translate into improved cognitive function and mental clarity in daily life.
4. **Boosted Self-Confidence**: As individuals progress in their Pilates practice and notice improvements in their strength, flexibility, and overall fitness, they often experience a boost in self-confidence and body image.

Introduction to the Pilates Reformer

The Pilates Reformer is one of the most iconic pieces of equipment in the Pilates repertoire. Known for its versatility and ability to provide a full-body workout, the Reformer has revolutionized how Pilates is practiced, offering numerous benefits that enhance traditional mat exercises.

Description and Components of the Reformer Machine

The Pilates Reformer is a sophisticated piece of apparatus designed to facilitate a wide range of exercises that improve strength, flexibility, balance, and coordination. At first glance, the Reformer may appear complex, but its components are thoughtfully designed to work together harmoniously, allowing for controlled, precise movements.

1. The Carriage The central feature of the Reformer is the carriage, a padded, flat platform that moves back and forth along the frame of the machine. The carriage is where most exercises are performed, either seated, lying down, or kneeling. Its movement is smooth and controlled, thanks to a series of wheels or rollers that glide along tracks in the frame.

2. Springs Attached to the front end of the carriage are a set of springs of varying resistance levels. These springs can be adjusted to increase or decrease the resistance, providing tailored challenges for different exercises and fitness levels. The resistance offered by the springs helps to build strength and muscle endurance.

3. Footbar At the front end of the Reformer is the footbar, a padded bar that can be adjusted to different heights and angles. The footbar serves as a support for the feet or hands, depending on the exercise. It plays a crucial role in many Reformer exercises, providing a stable platform to push against and helping to align the body correctly.

4. Shoulder Blocks The carriage features shoulder blocks, which are padded supports located near the head of the carriage. These blocks help to keep the body stable and aligned during exercises, especially when pushing or pulling against the resistance of the springs.

5. Straps and Ropes The Reformer is equipped with a set of straps and ropes attached to pulleys. These straps can be used for exercises involving the arms or legs, allowing for a greater range of motion and variety in the workout. The length of the ropes can be adjusted to modify the range and intensity of exercises.

6. Headrest The headrest is an adjustable, padded support for the head, providing comfort and proper alignment during exercises performed lying down on the carriage.

7. Frame and Stand The entire apparatus is supported by a sturdy frame, which may be set on a stand to raise it off the floor. This elevated position can make it easier to mount and dismount the machine, and can also offer additional exercise variations.

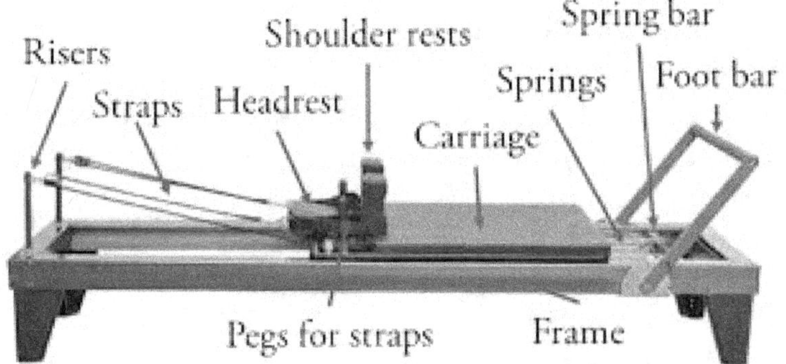

How the Reformer Enhances Pilates Practice

The Pilates Reformer enhances Pilates practice by introducing resistance, support, and versatility, transforming traditional mat exercises into more dynamic and challenging workouts.

1. Resistance Training The adjustable springs on the Reformer provide varying levels of resistance, which can be tailored to individual needs and progressions. This resistance helps to build and tone muscles, improve endurance, and increase overall strength. Unlike traditional weightlifting, the resistance on the Reformer is smooth and controlled, reducing the risk of injury and ensuring proper muscle engagement.

2. Full-Body Workout The Reformer is designed to engage multiple muscle groups simultaneously, promoting balanced muscle development and coordination. Exercises on the Reformer often target the core, arms, legs, and back, providing a comprehensive workout that enhances overall fitness and functionality.

3. Improved Flexibility and Range of Motion The Reformer allows for a greater range of motion compared to mat exercises alone. The carriage's movement and the adjustable straps enable deeper stretches and more fluid movements, helping to improve flexibility and joint mobility. This is particularly beneficial for individuals recovering from injuries or those with limited flexibility.

4. Enhanced Core Strength Core strength is a fundamental aspect of Pilates, and the Reformer intensifies core engagement through various exercises. The instability of the moving carriage requires constant activation of the core muscles to maintain balance and control, leading to a stronger and more stable core.

5. Precision and Alignment The design of the Reformer, with its adjustable components and supportive features, promotes proper body alignment and form. The footbar, shoulder blocks, and headrest help ensure that the body is correctly positioned during exercises, reducing the risk of injury and enhancing the effectiveness of each movement.

6. Versatility and Adaptability One of the greatest advantages of the Reformer is its versatility. The machine can be used for a wide variety of exercises, from gentle stretches to intense strength training. It can be adapted to suit different fitness levels, physical abilities, and rehabilitation needs, making it accessible to a broad range of individuals.

7. Mental Focus and Mind-Body Connection Like all Pilates practice, working on the Reformer requires concentration and mental focus. The precision and control needed for Reformer exercises foster a strong mind-body connection, enhancing body awareness and promoting mindfulness.

Part 1: Understanding Pilates Principles

Chapter 1: The Core Pilates Principles

Concentration

Focusing on Body Movements and Mind-Body Connection

Concentration is a fundamental principle of Pilates, and it is integral to the practice's effectiveness. This principle emphasizes the importance of focusing intently on each movement, ensuring that exercises are performed with precision and control. Concentration fosters a strong mind-body connection, which is essential for achieving the full benefits of Pilates.

1. Mindful Movement Concentration in Pilates means being fully present in the moment and aware of every part of your body. This mindfulness ensures that each exercise is executed with intention and accuracy, maximizing its effectiveness. By focusing on the movement, you can better control your muscles and maintain proper form, reducing the risk of injury and enhancing the overall quality of your workout.

2. Enhancing Body Awareness Developing body awareness is a key aspect of concentration. By paying close attention to how your body feels and moves, you can identify any imbalances or areas of tension. This awareness allows you to make necessary adjustments to your posture and alignment, leading to more efficient and effective movements. Over time, this heightened awareness helps improve coordination, balance, and overall physical performance.

3. Mental Focus and Clarity Pilates encourages mental focus and clarity by requiring you to concentrate on each exercise. This mental engagement not only improves your ability to perform the movements correctly but also provides a form of mental relaxation. The focus required during Pilates can help reduce stress and anxiety, as it allows you to take a break from the demands of daily life and concentrate solely on your body and breath.

4. Building a Strong Mind-Body Connection The mind-body connection is a central concept in Pilates, and concentration is crucial to developing this connection. By focusing on your breath, muscle engagement, and movement patterns, you create a deeper connection between your mind and body. This connection enhances your ability to control your movements and engage the appropriate muscles, leading to more efficient and effective workouts.

5. Improving Precision and Control Concentration helps improve precision and control, which are essential for performing Pilates exercises correctly. Each movement in Pilates is designed to be precise and controlled, targeting specific muscle groups and promoting balanced muscle development. By concentrating on the details of each exercise, you can ensure that you are performing them accurately, which maximizes their benefits and minimizes the risk of injury.

6. Cultivating Discipline and Patience The principle of concentration also cultivates discipline and patience. Pilates is not about rushing through exercises or achieving immediate results. Instead, it is a practice that requires consistent effort and focus. By concentrating on each movement and taking the time to perform exercises correctly, you develop the discipline and patience needed to progress in your practice and achieve long-term results.

7. Enhancing the Pilates Experience Concentration enhances the overall Pilates experience by making each session more engaging and rewarding. When you are fully focused on your movements, you can experience the subtleties and nuances of each exercise, which can make your practice more enjoyable and fulfilling. This focus also helps you stay motivated and committed to your Pilates journey, as you can see and feel the benefits of your efforts.

Practical Tips for Enhancing Concentration in Pilates:

- **Breath Awareness:** Focus on your breath throughout each exercise. Use your breath to guide your movements and help maintain a steady rhythm.
- **Set Intentions:** Begin each Pilates session by setting an intention for your practice. This intention can help you stay focused and motivated.
- **Eliminate Distractions:** Create a quiet and calm environment for your Pilates practice.

Turn off electronic devices and eliminate any distractions that could take your focus away from your movements.

- **Visualize Movements:** Visualize each movement before performing it. This mental rehearsal can help improve your concentration and execution of the exercise.
- **Use Cues:** Pay attention to cues from your instructor or from instructional materials. These cues can help you focus on specific aspects of each movement and improve your technique

Control

Importance of Controlled Movements for Effective Practice

Control is a central principle of Pilates, emphasizing the need for precision and careful execution of each movement. Joseph Pilates, the founder of the Pilates method, originally named his method "Contrology" to highlight the significance of controlled movements. The emphasis on control ensures that exercises are performed correctly, safely, and effectively, maximizing their benefits and minimizing the risk of injury.

1. Precision and Quality Over Quantity In Pilates, the quality of movement is more important than the quantity. Controlled movements ensure that each exercise is executed with precision, targeting specific muscle groups and promoting balanced muscle development. This focus on precision enhances the effectiveness of the workout, as it allows for maximum muscle engagement and proper alignment.

2. Preventing Injury Controlled movements are crucial for injury prevention. By performing exercises with control, you reduce the risk of sudden, jerky motions that can strain muscles or joints. Control allows for smooth, deliberate movements that protect the body from unnecessary stress and help maintain proper form.

3. Enhancing Muscle Engagement Control ensures that the correct muscles are engaged during each exercise. This targeted muscle engagement promotes balanced muscle development and prevents overuse or underuse of certain muscle groups. Controlled movements also help activate stabilizing muscles, which are essential for maintaining proper posture and alignment.

4. Building Strength and Endurance Controlled movements contribute to building strength and endurance. By performing exercises slowly and deliberately, you increase the time muscles are under tension, which enhances muscle strength and endurance. Control also allows for a greater range of motion, which helps improve flexibility and mobility.

5. Improving Focus and Mind-Body Connection Control enhances focus and the mind-body connection. Concentrating on controlled movements requires mental engagement, which helps create a deeper connection between the mind and body. This connection improves body awareness, coordination, and overall physical performance.

6. Promoting Efficiency and Effectiveness Controlled movements promote efficiency and effectiveness in your Pilates practice. By performing exercises with control, you ensure that each movement is purposeful and contributes to your fitness goals. This efficiency maximizes the benefits of your workout and helps you achieve desired results more effectively.

Practical Tips for Enhancing Control in Pilates:

- **Focus on Breathing:** Use your breath to guide and control your movements. Inhale to prepare for a movement and exhale as you execute it, ensuring smooth and controlled transitions.
- **Move Slowly and Deliberately:** Perform exercises slowly and deliberately, focusing on the quality of each movement rather than rushing through repetitions.
- **Engage Your Core:** Maintain core engagement throughout each exercise to support controlled movements and proper alignment.
- **Use Visual Cues:** Visualize the movement before performing it, and imagine the muscles working to control the motion.
- **Practice Mindfulness:** Stay present and mindful during your practice, focusing on each movement and maintaining control throughout the exercise.

Centering

Engaging the Core and Maintaining Balance

Centering is another fundamental principle of Pilates, focusing on the engagement of the core muscles and the maintenance of balance. The "center" or "core" refers to the muscles of the abdomen, lower back, hips, and pelvis. These muscles form the powerhouse of the body, providing stability and support for all movements.

1. Core Engagement for Stability Engaging the core muscles is essential for stability and balance. The core acts as a foundation for all movements, providing a stable base from which the limbs can move freely. A strong and engaged core helps maintain proper alignment and posture, reducing the risk of injury and enhancing overall physical performance.

2. Enhancing Balance and Coordination Centering promotes balance and coordination. By engaging the core, you improve your ability to control movements and maintain balance, both in static positions and dynamic exercises. This improved balance and coordination translate to better performance in other physical activities and daily tasks.

3. Supporting Proper Posture A strong core supports proper posture. Engaging the core muscles helps maintain a neutral spine alignment, preventing slouching or excessive curvature. Good posture is essential for overall health, as it reduces strain on the spine and prevents musculoskeletal issues.

4. Improving Efficiency of Movement Centering enhances the efficiency of movement. A strong and engaged core allows for more efficient transfer of energy through the body, making movements smoother and more coordinated. This efficiency reduces unnecessary strain on other muscle groups and promotes more effective workouts.

5. Reducing the Risk of Injury Engaging the core muscles reduces the risk of injury. A stable core provides better support for the spine and pelvis, protecting them from excessive stress and strain. This stability is especially important during dynamic movements and weight-bearing exercises.

6. Promoting Overall Physical Health Centering promotes overall physical health and well-being. A strong core supports better movement patterns, enhances athletic performance, and reduces the risk of chronic pain and injury. Core engagement is also beneficial for activities of daily living, making movements more efficient and reducing the risk of falls or injuries.

Practical Tips for Enhancing Centering in Pilates:

- **Engage Your Core:** Focus on engaging your core muscles during each exercise. Imagine pulling your navel toward your spine to activate the deep abdominal muscles.

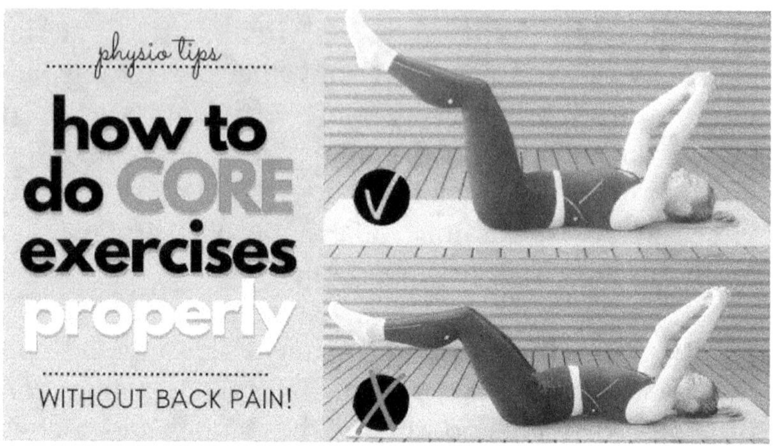

- **Maintain Neutral Spine:** Ensure that your spine remains in a neutral position, avoiding excessive arching or rounding of the back.
- **Use Breath to Support Core Engagement:** Use your breath to support core engagement. Inhale to prepare and exhale to engage the core and stabilize the body.
- **Practice Balance Exercises:** Incorporate balance exercises into your routine to improve core stability and coordination.
- **Visualize the Core:** Visualize the core as the powerhouse of your body, providing support and stability for all movements.

Flow

Creating Smooth, Continuous Movements

Flow, also known as fluidity, is a core principle of Pilates that emphasizes the importance of creating smooth, continuous movements during exercise. This principle aims to make each transition seamless, promoting efficiency and grace in motion.

1. Enhancing Coordination and Grace Flow encourages the development of coordination and grace in movement. By focusing on smooth transitions, you can achieve a more harmonious and fluid practice, which not only looks elegant but also feels more natural and enjoyable.

2. Improving Movement Efficiency Smooth, continuous movements are more efficient than jerky, disjointed ones. Flow ensures that energy is conserved and distributed evenly throughout the body, making each exercise more effective and less tiring. This efficiency helps in maintaining stamina and reducing fatigue during workouts.

3. Reducing Risk of Injury Flow reduces the risk of injury by minimizing abrupt, uncontrolled movements that can strain muscles and joints. By practicing smooth transitions, you can maintain better control over your body, ensuring that each movement is performed safely and with proper alignment.

4. Promoting Mind-Body Connection Flow enhances the mind-body connection by requiring continuous mental focus. Concentrating on creating smooth transitions helps deepen your awareness of how your body moves, improving overall body awareness and control. This heightened awareness can translate into better performance in other physical activities and daily tasks.

5. Supporting Cardiovascular Health Continuous movement in Pilates can provide a low-impact cardiovascular workout. Flow keeps your heart rate elevated without placing undue stress on your joints, making it an excellent option for improving cardiovascular health in a safe and controlled manner.

Practical Tips for Enhancing Flow in Pilates:

- **Focus on Transitions:** Pay attention to how you move from one exercise to the next. Aim for smooth, seamless transitions without stopping or jerking.
- **Maintain a Steady Pace:** Keep a steady, consistent pace throughout your workout. Avoid rushing through exercises or lingering too long in any one position.
- **Use Breath to Guide Movement:** Coordinate your breath with your movements to create a natural rhythm. Inhale to prepare and exhale to execute, allowing your breath to support smooth transitions.
- **Stay Mindful:** Concentrate on the quality of your movements. Visualize the flow of energy through your body, ensuring that each movement is purposeful and controlled.
- **Practice Regularly:** Like any skill, flow improves with practice. Incorporate flow-focused exercises into your regular Pilates routine to develop smoother, more fluid movements over time.

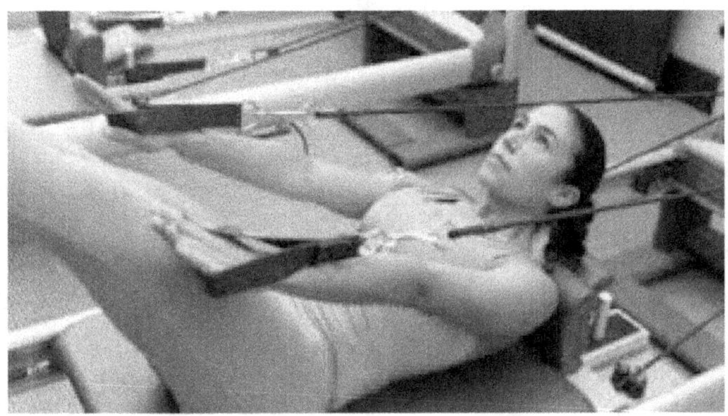

Precision

Performing Exercises with Accuracy and Attention to Detail

Precision is a fundamental principle of Pilates that involves performing exercises with accuracy and meticulous attention to detail. This principle ensures that each movement is executed correctly, maximizing the effectiveness of the exercise and minimizing the risk of injury.

1. Maximizing Effectiveness Precision ensures that each exercise targets the intended muscle groups effectively. By performing movements accurately, you can engage the correct muscles, enhancing the overall effectiveness of your workout. This focus on precision leads to better results in terms of strength, flexibility, and muscle tone.

2. Enhancing Muscle Control Precision helps develop muscle control and coordination. By concentrating on detailed execution, you can improve your ability to control and isolate specific muscles. This control is essential for achieving balanced muscle development and preventing muscle imbalances that can lead to injury.

3. Preventing Injury Performing exercises with precision reduces the risk of injury. Accurate movements ensure proper alignment and technique, minimizing the strain on muscles, joints, and ligaments. This attention to detail helps protect your body from unnecessary stress and injury.

4. Promoting Mind-Body Connection Precision enhances the mind-body connection by requiring focused attention on each movement. This focus helps deepen your awareness of how your body moves and responds to different exercises. The increased body awareness improves overall coordination and control.

5. Supporting Progression Precision is essential for progression in Pilates. As you master the basics with accuracy, you can gradually progress to more advanced exercises with confidence. This step-by-step approach ensures that you build a strong foundation before moving on to more challenging movements.

Practical Tips for Enhancing Precision in Pilates:

- **Follow Instructions Carefully:** Pay close attention to the instructions provided for each exercise. Follow the steps precisely to ensure correct execution.
- **Use Visual Cues:** Visualize the movement and the muscles involved before performing the

exercise. This mental preparation can help you execute the movement more accurately.

- **Practice Mindfulness:** Stay present and focused during your practice. Concentrate on the details of each movement, ensuring that you perform it with precision.
- **Seek Feedback:** Work with a qualified instructor or use mirrors to check your form. Feedback can help you identify and correct any errors in your technique.
- **Take Your Time:** Avoid rushing through exercises. Take your time to perform each movement with care and attention to detail.

Breathing

Proper Breathing Techniques to Support Movement and Relaxation

Breathing is a cornerstone of the Pilates method, intricately woven into every exercise to enhance movement, support relaxation, and promote overall well-being. Proper breathing techniques in Pilates not only facilitate better oxygen flow but also help to synchronize the mind and body, ensuring that each movement is executed with precision and control. Understanding and mastering Pilates breathing can significantly elevate the quality and effectiveness of your practice.

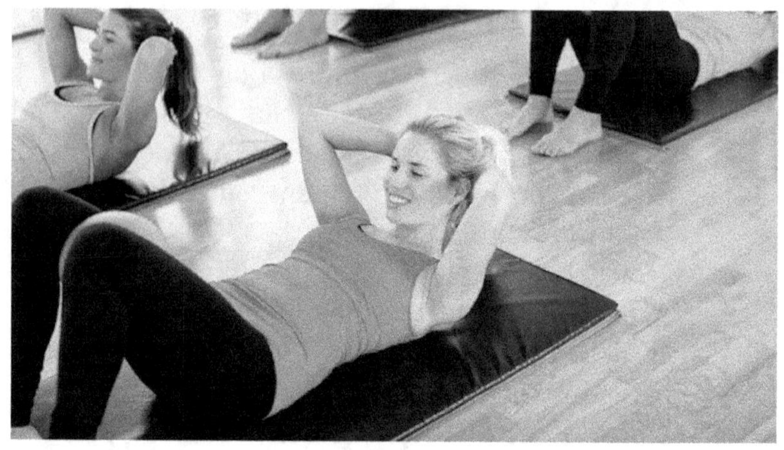

1. The Importance of Breath in Pilates

Breathing in Pilates is not just a background activity; it is a dynamic component that influences the entire practice. Joseph Pilates, the founder of the method, believed that proper breathing was essential for cleansing the bloodstream and invigorating the body. By incorporating specific breathing patterns, Pilates exercises aim to optimize oxygen delivery to muscles, enhance concentration, and support the core muscles, which are central to many Pilates movements.

2. Types of Breathing in Pilates

There are two primary types of breathing techniques in Pilates: lateral (or ribcage) breathing and diaphragmatic breathing.

Lateral Breathing:

- **Technique:** Lateral breathing involves expanding the ribcage sideways on inhalation and contracting it on exhalation. This method allows practitioners to keep the abdominal muscles engaged throughout the exercise.

- **Benefits:** By expanding the ribs laterally, you can maintain a stable core while still allowing deep, full breaths. This technique is particularly beneficial during exercises that require strong core engagement and stability.

Diaphragmatic Breathing:

- **Technique:** Diaphragmatic breathing, often referred to as "belly breathing," involves deep inhalations that expand the diaphragm and fill the lower lungs, followed by full exhalations.
- **Benefits:** This type of breathing promotes relaxation, reduces stress, and enhances oxygen exchange. It is particularly useful during warm-ups, cool-downs, and less intense exercises where deep relaxation is desired.

3. Synchronizing Breath with Movement

In Pilates, each movement is synchronized with breath to create a fluid and controlled practice. This synchronization enhances the efficiency and effectiveness of the exercises, ensuring that movements are performed with the appropriate intensity and support. Here are some guidelines for coordinating breath with movement:

- **Inhale to Prepare:** Inhale deeply to prepare for the movement, filling the lungs with oxygen and setting the stage for a controlled execution.

- **Exhale on Effort:** Exhale during the most challenging phase of the movement, such as lifting, twisting, or pressing. This helps to engage the core muscles and provides additional stability and power.
- **Inhale to Lengthen:** Use inhalation to create space and length in the body, especially during stretching or elongation movements.
- **Exhale to Deepen:** Exhale to deepen the contraction or stretch, allowing for greater control and intensity in the movement.

4. Benefits of Proper Breathing in Pilates

Enhanced Core Stability: Proper breathing techniques, particularly lateral breathing, help maintain core stability throughout the practice. By keeping the abdominal muscles engaged, practitioners can perform movements with greater control and precision.

Improved Concentration and Mindfulness: Focusing on breath enhances mental clarity and mindfulness. This heightened awareness allows practitioners to fully engage in the present moment, improving the overall quality of the workout.

Increased Oxygenation and Endurance: Effective breathing ensures that muscles receive adequate oxygen, reducing fatigue and increasing endurance. This is particularly important in Pilates, where sustained muscle engagement is often required.

Stress Reduction and Relaxation: Deep, controlled breathing promotes relaxation and reduces stress. This not only benefits physical health but also enhances mental well-being, creating a more holistic approach to fitness.

5. Practical Tips for Mastering Pilates Breathing

- **Practice Regularly:** Like any skill, mastering Pilates breathing requires regular practice. Incorporate breathing exercises into your daily routine to build familiarity and control.
- **Stay Mindful:** Focus on your breath during each exercise, paying attention to how it supports and enhances your movements.
- **Seek Guidance:** If you're new to Pilates, consider working with a certified instructor who can provide personalized guidance on proper breathing techniques.
- **Use Visualization:** Visualize the breath filling your body and supporting your movements. This can help you connect more deeply with the breath and its role in your practice.

Chapter 2: Applying Principles to Reformer Workouts

Enhancing Reformer Exercises with Core Principles

The Pilates Reformer is an innovative piece of equipment designed to take your Pilates practice to the next level. By incorporating the core principles of Pilates—Concentration, Control, Centering, Flow, Precision, and Breathing—you can enhance the effectiveness and efficiency of your Reformer workouts. Understanding how these principles apply to Reformer exercises is crucial for achieving the best results and experiencing the full benefits of Pilates.

How Principles Translate to Reformer Workouts

1. Concentration: Focused Engagement

Concentration is the foundation of every Pilates exercise. It involves directing your mental focus to the movement, ensuring that each action is deliberate and purposeful. On the Reformer, concentration is key to maintaining proper form and alignment, which is crucial for both effectiveness and safety.

- **Application:** Before beginning any Reformer exercise, take a moment to mentally prepare. Focus on the specific muscles you intend to engage and visualize the movement. During the exercise, maintain this mental focus to ensure that each movement is precise and controlled.

- **Example:** In the "Footwork" series, concentrate on the alignment of your feet, legs, and hips, ensuring that each movement is smooth and controlled. Focus on the sensation of your muscles working against the resistance of the springs.

2. Control: Mastery Over Movement

Control is about managing the precision and quality of each movement, avoiding any jerky or uncontrolled motions. The Reformer, with its adjustable springs and sliding carriage, demands a high level of control to perform exercises effectively.

- **Application:** Use the Reformer's springs to control the intensity and pace of your movements. Focus on slow, deliberate actions that allow you to maintain control throughout the entire range of motion.
- **Example:** In the "Elephant" exercise, control the movement of the carriage as you push it out and draw it back in. Ensure that your core is engaged and that you are moving smoothly without any sudden or jarring motions.

3. Centering: Engaging the Core

Centering refers to the activation and engagement of the core muscles, which are the foundation of Pilates exercises. The Reformer provides an excellent platform for deep core engagement, as many exercises require stabilization against the resistance of the springs.

- **Application:** Engage your abdominal muscles, lower back, and pelvic floor throughout each exercise. Use your core to stabilize your body and support your movements, especially when working against the resistance of the springs.
- **Example:** During "The Hundred," focus on drawing your navel toward your spine and maintaining a strong, supported core while you pump your arms.

4. Flow: Creating Smooth Transitions

Flow involves creating smooth, continuous movements between exercises, maintaining a seamless and uninterrupted workout. The Reformer's sliding carriage facilitates fluid transitions, allowing you to maintain a steady rhythm throughout your practice.

- **Application:** Move with intention and fluidity from one exercise to the next. Avoid any pauses or breaks that disrupt the flow, and use controlled breathing to maintain a steady rhythm.
- **Example:** Transitioning from "Footwork" to "The Hundred" should be done smoothly, maintaining the momentum and avoiding any abrupt changes in pace or intensity.

5. Precision: Attention to Detail

Precision involves executing each movement with accuracy, focusing on alignment and correct technique. The Reformer's adjustable springs and sliding carriage allow for precise adjustments and fine-tuning of each exercise.

- **Application:** Pay attention to the details of each movement, including alignment, form, and range of motion. Make necessary adjustments to the springs and your body position to ensure that each exercise is performed with exactitude.
- **Example:** In the "Short Box Series," focus on precise movements, ensuring that your spine remains in alignment and that you are using the correct amount of resistance to challenge your muscles effectively.

6. Breathing: Synchronizing Breath with Movement

Breathing in Pilates involves coordinating your breath with your movements to support and enhance performance. Proper breathing techniques help facilitate movement, improve oxygenation, and support relaxation.

- **Application:** Inhale to prepare for the movement and exhale during the exertion phase. Use breathing to help guide your movements, maintain core engagement, and support relaxation during exercises.
- **Example:** In the "Leg Circles" exercise, inhale as you prepare to move your leg and exhale as you execute the circle, maintaining steady and controlled breathing throughout.

Integrating Core Principles in Reformer Workouts

To integrate these core principles into your Reformer workouts, consider the following strategies:

- **Mindful Practice:** Approach each Reformer session with mindfulness, fully engaging both your body and mind in the exercise. This will help you to internalize the principles and apply them effectively.
- **Progressive Learning:** Start with basic exercises to build a strong foundation, gradually incorporating more complex movements as you become more proficient in applying the core principles.
- **Feedback and Adjustment:** Pay close attention to your body's feedback during exercises. Make adjustments to your form, resistance, and breathing as needed to maintain alignment and control.
- **Consistency:** Regular practice is key to mastering the core principles. Consistency in your Reformer workouts will help reinforce these principles and improve your overall performance.

Examples of Principle-Driven Exercises

Applying the core principles of Pilates to specific Reformer exercises allows practitioners to experience the full benefits of this powerful fitness modality. By focusing on Concentration, Control, Centering, Flow, Precision, and Breathing, you can perform exercises more effectively and safely. Here are examples of Reformer exercises that demonstrate each principle:

1. Concentration: Footwork Series

The Footwork Series on the Reformer is an excellent example of how concentration can enhance an exercise. This series involves pushing the carriage away from the footbar using your legs, focusing on different positions of the feet (heels, toes, and arches).

- **Execution:**
  - **Heels on Footbar:** Lie on your back with your heels on the footbar, legs parallel. Inhale to prepare, then exhale as you press the carriage away, straightening your legs. Inhale as you bend your knees to return.
  - **Toes on Footbar:** Place the balls of your feet on the footbar, heels lifted. Repeat the pressing and returning motion, concentrating on maintaining a steady and controlled movement.
  - **Arches on Footbar:** Place the arches of your feet on the footbar and repeat the exercise.
- **Concentration:** Focus on the alignment of your legs and feet, ensuring that your knees and toes point in the same direction. Maintain mental awareness of your core engagement and the smooth movement of the carriage.

2. Control: Elephant

The Elephant exercise emphasizes control, particularly in maintaining a stable and controlled movement of the carriage while engaging the core.

- **Execution:**
  - Stand on the Reformer with your feet flat against the shoulder rests and hands on the footbar. Your body should form an inverted V-shape.
  - Inhale to prepare, then exhale as you press the carriage back with your feet, extending your legs while maintaining the V-shape.
  - Inhale as you draw the carriage back in, using your core muscles to control the movement.
- **Control:** Focus on controlling the movement of the carriage with your core and leg muscles, avoiding any jerky or uncontrolled motions. Keep your upper body stable and your spine neutral.

3. Centering: The Hundred

The Hundred is a classic Pilates exercise that engages the core muscles intensely. Performing this exercise on the Reformer adds an additional challenge with the use of resistance.

- **Execution:**
  - Lie on your back with your legs in tabletop position and your hands holding

the straps. Lift your head, neck, and shoulders off the carriage.
  - o Inhale to prepare, then exhale as you extend your legs to a 45-degree angle and pump your arms up and down while maintaining core engagement.
  - o Perform ten breaths (inhale for five counts, exhale for five counts) to complete 100 arm pumps.
- **Centering:** Engage your core muscles throughout the exercise, keeping your lower back pressed into the carriage. Focus on maintaining a stable torso and controlled breathing.

4. Flow: Coordination

The Coordination exercise on the Reformer highlights the principle of flow by requiring smooth and continuous movements. This exercise combines arm and leg movements in a coordinated, flowing sequence.

- **Execution:**
  - o Lie on your back with your legs in tabletop position and your hands holding the straps.
  - o Inhale to prepare, then exhale as you extend your arms and legs simultaneously, straightening them in front of you.

- Inhale as you open your legs to shoulder-width apart, then exhale as you bring them back together.
  - Bend your elbows and knees simultaneously to return to the starting position.
- **Flow:** Focus on creating smooth, continuous movements throughout the exercise, transitioning seamlessly from one phase to the next. Maintain a steady rhythm and avoid any pauses.

5. Precision: Short Box Series

The Short Box Series involves a series of exercises performed while sitting on the Reformer box. These exercises emphasize precision in movement and alignment.

- **Execution:**
  - Sit on the Reformer box with your feet secured under the foot strap. Hold a pole or your arms across your chest.
  - Perform exercises such as the "Round Back," "Flat Back," "Side-to-Side," and "Twist and Reach," focusing on precise movements and alignment.
  - For the "Round Back," inhale to prepare, then exhale as you roll back, articulating your spine one vertebra at a time. Inhale as you roll back up to the starting position.

- **Precision:** Pay attention to the alignment of your spine and pelvis, ensuring that each movement is precise and controlled. Focus on the exact execution of each phase of the exercise.

6. Breathing: Leg Circles

Leg Circles on the Reformer integrate breathing with movement, enhancing the flow and effectiveness of the exercise.

- **Execution:**
  - Lie on your back with your legs extended toward the ceiling, holding the straps.
  - Inhale to prepare, then exhale as you circle your legs outward and downward in a controlled motion.
  - Inhale as you bring your legs back up to the starting position, maintaining a smooth and continuous flow.
- **Breathing:** Coordinate your breathing with your leg movements, exhaling as you lower your legs and inhaling as you raise them. Focus on maintaining a steady and rhythmic breath throughout the exercise.

Integrating Principle-Driven Exercises into Your Routine

By incorporating these principle-driven exercises into your Reformer routine, you can enhance the effectiveness and enjoyment of your Pilates practice.

Each exercise emphasizes one or more of the core principles, helping you develop a deeper understanding and mastery of Pilates. Remember to approach each exercise with mindfulness, focusing on the principles of Concentration, Control, Centering, Flow, Precision, and Breathing to achieve the best results.

Part 2: Building a Strong Foundation

Chapter 3: Basic Reformer Exercises

Introduction to Basic Reformer Exercises

Starting with basic exercises is essential for anyone new to the Pilates Reformer. These foundational movements help you understand how to use the Reformer, develop body awareness, and build the strength and stability necessary for more advanced exercises. This chapter will guide you through essential Reformer exercises, detailing their execution, benefits, and modifications to ensure a safe and effective practice.

1. Footwork Series

The Footwork Series is often the starting point in a Reformer workout, focusing on the legs and core while warming up the body.

- **Execution:**
    - **Position:** Lie on your back with your head on the headrest, feet on the footbar.
    - **Heels Parallel:** Place heels on the footbar, hip-width apart. Inhale to prepare, exhale as you press the carriage away by extending your legs, then inhale to return.
    - **Toes Parallel:** Place the balls of your feet on the footbar, heels lifted. Perform

the same pressing motion, focusing on controlled movement.

- o **Heels Together, Toes Apart:** Create a small V-shape with your feet, heels together and toes apart. Press away and return, engaging inner thighs.
- o **Wide Heels and Toes:** Place feet wider on the footbar, either on heels or balls of feet, and repeat the pressing motion.
- **Benefits:** Strengthens leg muscles, improves joint mobility, warms up the body, and prepares for more challenging exercises.
- **Modifications:** Adjust the spring tension based on your fitness level. For beginners, start with lighter resistance.

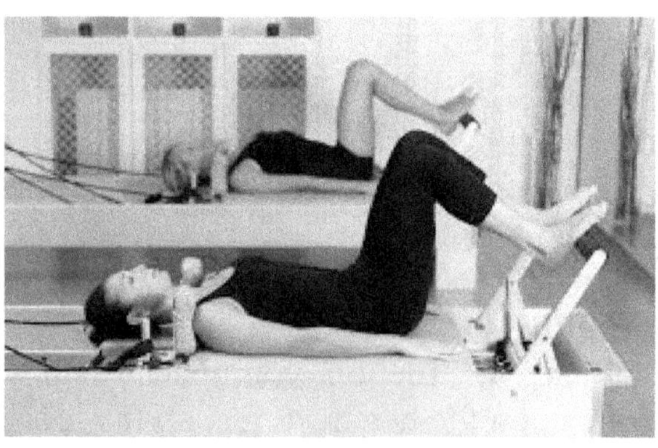

2. The Hundred

The Hundred is a core-centric exercise that also warms up the body and improves circulation.

- **Execution:**

- o **Position:** Lie on your back with your legs in tabletop position and hands holding the straps.
- o **Movement:** Lift your head, neck, and shoulders off the carriage. Extend your legs to a 45-degree angle. Pump your arms up and down vigorously, inhaling for five counts and exhaling for five counts, completing ten cycles.
- **Benefits:** Engages the core muscles, improves stamina, enhances coordination, and warms up the entire body.
- **Modifications:** Keep your legs bent at 90 degrees if extending them is too challenging. Lower your head if you experience neck discomfort.

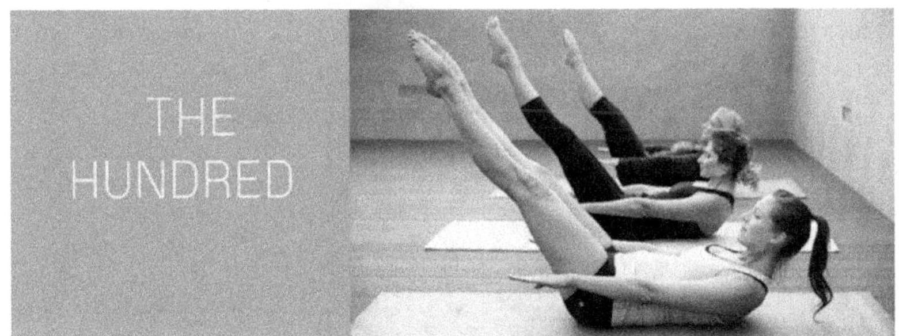

3. Leg Circles

Leg Circles enhance hip mobility and core stability.

- **Execution:**
  - o **Position:** Lie on your back with legs extended toward the ceiling, holding the straps.

- o **Movement:** Circle your legs outward and downward in a controlled motion. Complete a set of circles in one direction, then reverse.
- **Benefits:** Improves hip mobility, strengthens the core, and enhances coordination.
- **Modifications:** Bend your knees slightly if hamstring flexibility is limited. Decrease the range of motion to maintain control.

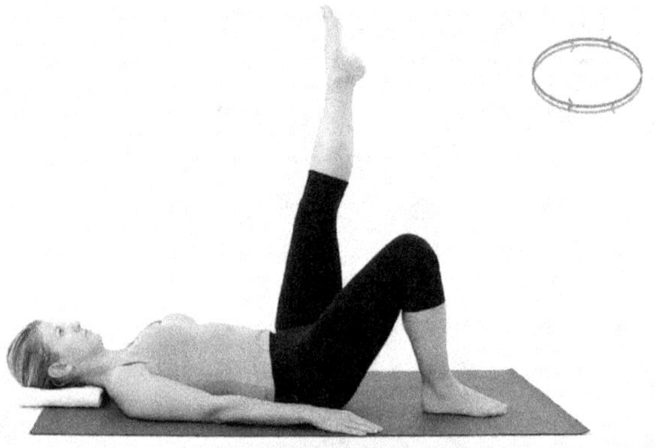

4. The Frog

The Frog exercise targets the inner thighs, glutes, and core.

- **Execution:**
    - o **Position:** Lie on your back with your head on the headrest, legs in tabletop position, feet in the straps.
    - o **Movement:** Extend your legs out at a 45-degree angle, then bend your knees and draw them back towards your

shoulders, resembling a frog's movement.

- **Benefits:** Strengthens inner thighs, glutes, and core, improves flexibility and coordination.
- **Modifications:** Adjust the spring tension for more or less resistance. Perform with bent knees if leg extension is challenging.

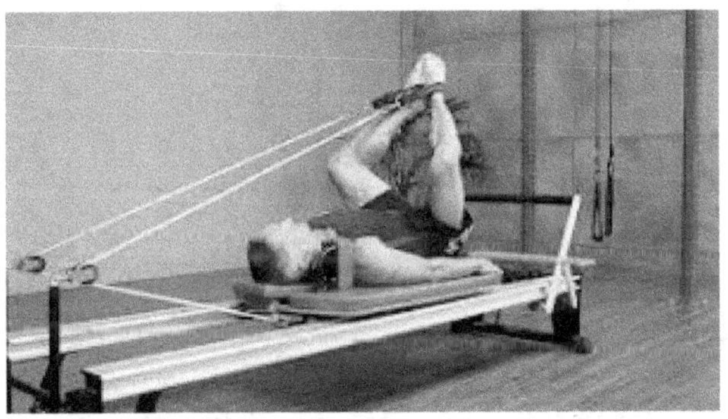

5. Arm Circles

Arm Circles strengthen the upper body while engaging the core.

- **Execution:**
    - **Position:** Lie on your back with legs bent or extended, arms holding the straps.
    - **Movement:** Circle your arms outward and downward in a controlled manner, then reverse the direction.
- **Benefits:** Strengthens shoulders, arms, and core, enhances upper body mobility.

- **Modifications:** Reduce the range of motion or perform with lighter resistance if shoulder mobility is limited.

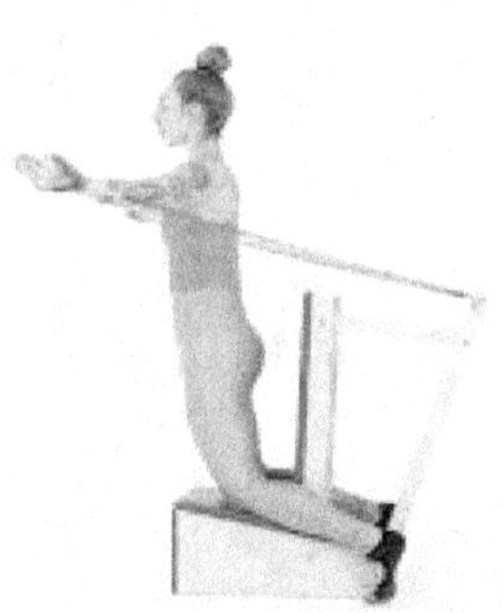

6. Elephant

The Elephant exercise focuses on hamstring flexibility and core strength.

- **Execution:**
    - **Position:** Stand on the Reformer with feet against the shoulder rests, hands on the footbar.
    - **Movement:** Form an inverted V-shape with your body. Press the carriage back with your feet, then draw it forward using your core.
- **Benefits:** Stretches hamstrings, strengthens the core, and improves balance.
- **Modifications:** Keep a slight bend in your knees if hamstring flexibility is limited. Reduce the range of motion to maintain control.

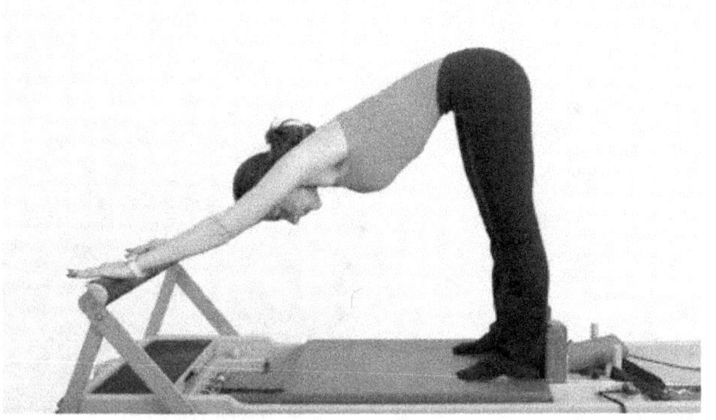

7. Knee Stretch Series

This series enhances core strength and leg power.

- **Execution:**
    - **Position:** Kneel on the carriage with hands on the footbar, knees under hips.
    - **Movement:** For "Round Back," tuck your pelvis and round your spine. For "Flat Back," maintain a neutral spine. Push the carriage back with your legs, then draw it forward using your core.
- **Benefits:** Strengthens core, legs, and glutes, improves posture.
- **Modifications:** Perform with lighter resistance or smaller range of motion if necessary.

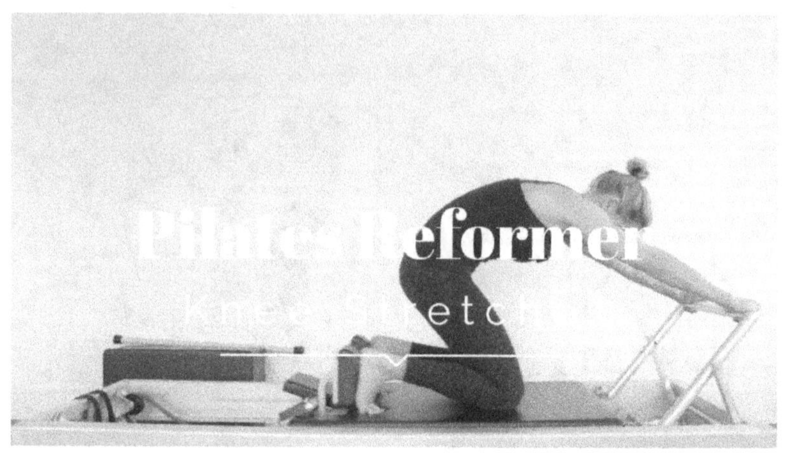

Conclusion: Building a Strong Foundation

Mastering these basic Reformer exercises lays the groundwork for more advanced movements. By focusing on proper form, controlled movement, and core engagement, you build the strength, stability, and confidence needed to progress in your Pilates practice. Remember to listen to your body, make necessary modifications, and practice regularly to achieve the best results.

Common Mistakes and How to Avoid Them

Tips for Proper Form and Technique

Ensuring proper form and technique in Reformer exercises is essential for effectiveness and injury prevention. Here are common mistakes and tips on how to avoid them:

1. Footwork Series

- **Mistake:** Allowing the knees to collapse inward or outward during the movement.
  - **Correction:** Focus on maintaining alignment from hips to knees to ankles. Engage inner thighs to keep knees tracking over the toes.
- **Mistake:** Using momentum to push the carriage.
  - **Correction:** Move slowly and with control, engaging muscles throughout the entire range of motion.

2. The Hundred

- **Mistake:** Straining the neck by lifting too high.
  - **Correction:** Keep your head and neck in a neutral position. If needed, place a small pillow under your head for support.
- **Mistake:** Pumping arms too vigorously, causing shoulder tension.
  - **Correction:** Pump arms with control, focusing on engaging the core and maintaining relaxed shoulders.

3. Leg Circles

- **Mistake:** Allowing the lower back to arch off the carriage.
  - **Correction:** Engage the core to keep the lower back pressed gently into the carriage. Limit the range of motion if necessary.

- **Mistake:** Moving the legs too quickly, losing control.
    - o **Correction:** Slow down the movement to ensure control and stability, focusing on smooth, circular motions.

4. The Frog

- **Mistake:** Letting the knees splay outward excessively.
    - o **Correction:** Keep the knees aligned with the shoulders and engage the inner thighs to control the movement.
- **Mistake:** Using the straps to pull legs back instead of engaging the core.
    - o **Correction:** Focus on using core muscles to draw legs back, maintaining control and alignment.

5. Arm Circles

- **Mistake:** Allowing the shoulders to lift towards the ears.
    - o **Correction:** Keep shoulders down and relaxed, focusing on engaging the shoulder blades and upper back muscles.
- **Mistake:** Moving arms too quickly, causing loss of control.
    - o **Correction:** Perform arm circles slowly and with precision, maintaining a steady, controlled pace.

6. Elephant

- **Mistake:** Rounding the back excessively, causing strain.
    - **Correction:** Maintain a neutral spine with a slight arch, focusing on engaging the core and lengthening the spine.
- **Mistake:** Pushing the carriage too far back, losing stability.
    - **Correction:** Limit the range of motion to maintain control and stability, focusing on smooth, controlled movements.

7. Knee Stretch Series

- **Round Back**
    - **Mistake:** Allowing the lower back to sag, losing the rounded position.
    - **Correction:** Keep the pelvis tucked and engage the core to maintain the rounded spine throughout the movement.
- **Flat Back**
    - **Mistake:** Arching the back excessively, causing strain.
    - **Correction:** Maintain a neutral spine with a strong core engagement. Focus on keeping the back flat and stable.

Chapter 4: Intermediate Reformer Exercises

As you advance in your Pilates journey, transitioning from basic to intermediate Reformer exercises is crucial for continued improvement and achieving a higher level of fitness. This chapter provides a comprehensive guide on how to progress your practice, introduces challenging exercises, and offers technique tips to enhance precision and effectiveness.

Progressing Your Practice

When and How to Move to Intermediate Exercises

1. Recognizing Readiness:

- **Consistency and Confidence:** Ensure you have a solid foundation in basic Reformer exercises, performing them consistently with confidence and correct form.
- **Core Strength and Stability:** Intermediate exercises demand greater core strength and stability. If you can maintain control and stability in basic exercises, you're ready to progress.
- **Instructor Guidance:** If possible, seek feedback from a certified Pilates instructor to confirm your readiness and receive personalized recommendations for progression.

2. Gradual Transition:

- **Introduce Gradually:** Incorporate one or two intermediate exercises into your routine at a time, ensuring you can perform them with control before adding more.
- **Modify as Needed:** Start with modifications or lighter resistance to master the movements before increasing intensity.
- **Listen to Your Body:** Pay attention to how your body responds to new challenges. Progress at a pace that feels right for you.

Challenging Exercises for Improvement

Short Spine Massage

- **Start Position:** Lie on your back with your head on the headrest and feet in the straps, legs extended at a 45-degree angle.
- **Movement:** Inhale to prepare. Exhale as you lift your hips off the carriage, bringing your legs overhead. Inhale as you bend your knees, drawing them towards your shoulders. Exhale as you roll down one vertebra at a time, extending your legs back to the starting position.
- **Benefits:** Enhances spinal flexibility, strengthens the core, and improves coordination.

Long Box Series

1. Pulling Straps I and II

- **Start Position:** Lie face down on the long box with your chest off the edge, holding the straps in your hands.
- **Movement (I):** Inhale to prepare. Exhale as you pull the straps down by your sides, lifting your chest and extending your spine. Inhale to return.
- **Movement (II):** Inhale to prepare. Exhale as you pull the straps outward in a T position, lifting your chest and extending your spine. Inhale to return.
- **Benefits:** Strengthens the back muscles, improves posture, and enhances shoulder stability.

2. Breaststroke

- **Start Position:** Lie face down on the long box with your chest off the edge, holding the straps in your hands.
- **Movement:** Inhale to prepare. Exhale as you circle your arms out to the sides and overhead while lifting your chest and extending your spine. Inhale to return.
- **Benefits:** Strengthens the upper back and shoulders, improves spinal extension and coordination.

Teaser

- **Start Position:** Sit on the Reformer with your feet against the shoulder rests, holding the straps in your hands.

- **Movement:** Inhale to prepare. Exhale as you roll down to a C-curve position, then lift your legs to a 45-degree angle and your upper body to a V position. Inhale to hold, then exhale to roll back down with control.
- **Benefits:** Strengthens the core, improves balance, and enhances coordination.

Technique Tips

Enhancing Precision and Effectiveness

1. Focus on Alignment:

- **Body Awareness:** Maintain awareness of your body alignment throughout each exercise. Ensure that your head, shoulders, hips, and feet are in proper alignment.
- **Core Engagement:** Continuously engage your core muscles to support your movements and maintain stability.

2. Control Your Movements:

- **Slow and Steady:** Perform each exercise slowly and with control. Avoid using momentum, which can compromise form and effectiveness.
- **Breath Coordination:** Coordinate your breath with your movements. Inhale to prepare, exhale during the exertion phase, and inhale during the return phase.

3. Adjust Resistance Appropriately:

- **Gradual Increase:** Gradually increase the resistance as your strength improves. Start with lighter resistance and focus on mastering the technique before adding more.
- **Challenge without Strain:** Choose a resistance level that challenges you but allows you to maintain proper form without strain.

4. Listen to Your Body:

- **Pain vs. Discomfort:** Differentiate between discomfort from challenging your muscles and pain from potential injury. If you experience pain, stop and reassess your form or resistance level.
- **Rest and Recovery:** Allow adequate rest and recovery between sessions to prevent overtraining and ensure continuous improvement.

5. Seek Professional Guidance:

- **Instructor Feedback:** Regularly consult with a certified Pilates instructor to receive feedback, refine your technique, and progress safely.
- **Personalized Modifications:** An instructor can provide personalized modifications and adjustments based on your individual needs and goals.

Part 4: Specialized Reformer Workouts

Chapter 6: Targeted Workouts

In this chapter, we delve into the art of customizing your Pilates Reformer workouts to target specific fitness goals. Whether you aim to enhance flexibility, build strength, increase endurance, or support rehabilitation, this guide offers detailed, goal-oriented routines to help you achieve optimal results.

Workouts for Specific Goals

Flexibility

Flexibility is a key component of overall fitness, contributing to better posture, reduced muscle tension, and a decreased risk of injury. Pilates Reformer workouts are exceptional for improving flexibility due to their focus on controlled, full-range movements. Here's how to design a Reformer workout to boost flexibility:

- **Dynamic Stretches:** Incorporate exercises like Leg Circles and Long Stretch to dynamically stretch and warm up the muscles, preparing them for deeper stretches.
- **Static Stretches:** Use exercises such as the Mermaid Stretch and the Seated Forward Fold to hold positions that lengthen the muscles and connective tissues.
- **Active Flexibility:** Include movements like the Elephant and the Swan, which combine strength and stretching to improve active flexibility.

Sample Flexibility Routine:

1. **Warm-Up:** Leg Circles (3 minutes)
2. **Dynamic Stretch:** Long Stretch (3 sets of 10 repetitions)
3. **Static Stretch:** Mermaid Stretch (2 sets of 30 seconds each side)
4. **Active Flexibility:** Elephant (2 sets of 8 repetitions)
5. **Cool Down:** Seated Forward Fold (2 sets of 30 seconds)

Strength

Strength training on the Reformer helps build muscle, improve bone density, and boost metabolic rate. Here's how to create a Reformer workout focused on strength:

- **Resistance Exercises:** Utilize the adjustable resistance of the Reformer to perform exercises such as Footwork and the Rowing Series, which target multiple muscle groups.
- **Isometric Holds:** Incorporate exercises like the Plank and the Shoulder Bridge, which involve holding positions to engage muscles without movement, enhancing strength.
- **Progressive Overload:** Gradually increase the resistance and complexity of exercises like the Teaser and the Elephant to continuously challenge and build muscle strength.

Sample Strength Routine:

1. **Warm-Up:** Footwork (3 sets of 10 repetitions)

2. **Resistance Exercise:** Rowing Series (3 sets of 10 repetitions each)
3. **Isometric Hold:** Plank (2 sets of 30 seconds)
4. **Progressive Overload:** Teaser (3 sets of 8 repetitions)
5. **Cool Down:** Shoulder Bridge (2 sets of 10 repetitions)

Endurance

Endurance workouts aim to improve cardiovascular fitness and muscular stamina, allowing you to sustain physical activity for longer periods. Here's how to design an endurance-focused Reformer routine:

- **Circuit Training:** Combine different exercises in a circuit format, such as Footwork, Jump Board, and Long Stretch, to keep the heart rate elevated.
- **Repetition Sets:** Perform high-repetition sets of exercises like Leg Circles and the Hundred to build muscular endurance.
- **Interval Training:** Integrate intervals of high-intensity exercises like Jump Board and Cross-Train Reformer with lower-intensity exercises to improve overall endurance.

Sample Endurance Routine:

1. **Warm-Up:** Footwork (2 sets of 15 repetitions)
2. **Circuit Training:** Jump Board (2 minutes), Long Stretch (2 minutes)

3. **Repetition Sets:** Leg Circles (3 sets of 20 repetitions each)
4. **Interval Training:** Jump Board (1 minute high intensity, 1 minute low intensity) – 3 cycles
5. **Cool Down:** Hundred (1 set of 100 repetitions)

Rehabilitation

The Pilates Reformer is widely used for rehabilitation due to its low-impact nature and ability to support and guide the body through controlled movements. Here's how to create a Reformer workout for rehabilitation:

- **Gentle Movements:** Start with gentle, controlled movements like Footwork and Leg Circles to reintroduce movement and improve range of motion.
- **Stabilization Exercises:** Focus on exercises that improve core stability and balance, such as the Pelvic Curl and Spine Stretch.
- **Gradual Progression:** Gradually increase the intensity and complexity of exercises like the Cat Stretch and Arm Circles as strength and mobility improve.

Sample Rehabilitation Routine:

1. **Warm-Up:** Footwork (2 sets of 10 repetitions)
2. **Gentle Movements:** Leg Circles (2 sets of 10 repetitions each side)
3. **Stabilization Exercise:** Pelvic Curl (3 sets of 8 repetitions)

4. **Gradual Progression:** Cat Stretch (2 sets of 10 repetitions), Arm Circles (2 sets of 10 repetitions each side)
5. **Cool Down:** Spine Stretch (2 sets of 8 repetitions)

Customizing Your Routine

Adapting Exercises to Meet Individual Fitness Goals

One of the greatest strengths of the Pilates Reformer is its versatility and adaptability, making it an excellent tool for customizing workouts to meet specific fitness goals. Whether you're looking to improve flexibility, build strength, enhance endurance, or support rehabilitation, the Reformer can be tailored to your unique needs and preferences. This section explores how to personalize your Pilates Reformer routine to achieve your fitness aspirations.

Understanding Your Fitness Goals

Before customizing your routine, it's essential to clearly define your fitness goals. Consider the following common objectives:

1. **Improving Flexibility**: You aim to enhance your range of motion and decrease muscle tightness.
2. **Building Strength**: Your goal is to increase muscle mass and improve overall strength.
3. **Enhancing Endurance**: You wish to boost cardiovascular fitness and muscular stamina.

4. **Supporting Rehabilitation**: You need to gently restore movement and strength after an injury.

Once you've identified your primary goal, you can begin to tailor your exercises to support these specific outcomes.

Adapting Exercises for Flexibility

Flexibility is crucial for overall physical health, helping to prevent injuries and improve performance in various activities. To tailor your Reformer routine for flexibility:

- **Focus on Dynamic Stretches**: Incorporate exercises that involve continuous movement to stretch muscles dynamically. Examples include the Leg Circles and the Long Stretch.
- **Integrate Static Stretches**: Add static stretches that allow you to hold positions and gradually deepen the stretch. Exercises like the Mermaid Stretch and the Seated Forward Fold are ideal.
- **Combine Strength and Flexibility**: Use exercises that build strength while enhancing flexibility, such as the Swan and the Elephant, which require controlled, stretching movements.

Sample Flexibility Routine:

1. **Warm-Up**: Leg Circles (3 minutes)
2. **Dynamic Stretch**: Long Stretch (3 sets of 10 repetitions)
3. **Static Stretch**: Mermaid Stretch (2 sets of 30 seconds each side)

4. **Strength and Flexibility**: Elephant (2 sets of 8 repetitions)
5. **Cool Down**: Seated Forward Fold (2 sets of 30 seconds)

Adapting Exercises for Strength

Strength training on the Reformer can significantly enhance muscle mass, bone density, and overall physical resilience. To customize your routine for strength:

- **Utilize Resistance**: Adjust the Reformer's resistance to challenge your muscles effectively. Exercises like Footwork and the Rowing Series can be performed with increased resistance to build strength.
- **Include Isometric Holds**: Integrate exercises that involve holding positions, such as the Plank and the Shoulder Bridge, to engage and strengthen muscles without movement.
- **Progressive Overload**: Gradually increase the resistance and complexity of exercises like the Teaser and the Elephant to continuously challenge your muscles.

Sample Strength Routine:

1. **Warm-Up**: Footwork (3 sets of 10 repetitions)
2. **Resistance Exercise**: Rowing Series (3 sets of 10 repetitions each)
3. **Isometric Hold**: Plank (2 sets of 30 seconds)
4. **Progressive Overload**: Teaser (3 sets of 8 repetitions)

5. **Cool Down**: Shoulder Bridge (2 sets of 10 repetitions)

Adapting Exercises for Endurance

Endurance training focuses on improving your ability to sustain physical activity over longer periods, benefiting both cardiovascular health and muscular stamina. To customize your routine for endurance:

- **Circuit Training**: Design your routine as a circuit, combining various exercises like Footwork, Jump Board, and Long Stretch to maintain an elevated heart rate.
- **High-Repetition Sets**: Perform exercises like Leg Circles and the Hundred with high repetitions to build endurance.
- **Interval Training**: Include intervals of high-intensity exercises such as the Jump Board and Cross-Train Reformer interspersed with lower-intensity exercises.

Sample Endurance Routine:

1. **Warm-Up**: Footwork (2 sets of 15 repetitions)
2. **Circuit Training**: Jump Board (2 minutes), Long Stretch (2 minutes)
3. **High-Repetition Sets**: Leg Circles (3 sets of 20 repetitions each)
4. **Interval Training**: Jump Board (1 minute high intensity, 1 minute low intensity) – 3 cycles
5. **Cool Down**: Hundred (1 set of 100 repetitions)

Adapting Exercises for Rehabilitation

Rehabilitation exercises on the Reformer are designed to gently restore movement and strength, making it an excellent tool for recovery from injury. To customize your routine for rehabilitation:

- **Start with Gentle Movements**: Begin with low-intensity, controlled exercises such as Footwork and Leg Circles to reintroduce movement and improve range of motion.
- **Focus on Stabilization**: Emphasize exercises that improve core stability and balance, like the Pelvic Curl and Spine Stretch.
- **Gradual Progression**: Slowly increase the intensity and complexity of exercises like the Cat Stretch and Arm Circles as your strength and mobility improve.

Sample Rehabilitation Routine:

1. **Warm-Up**: Footwork (2 sets of 10 repetitions)
2. **Gentle Movements**: Leg Circles (2 sets of 10 repetitions each side)
3. **Stabilization Exercise**: Pelvic Curl (3 sets of 8 repetitions)
4. **Gradual Progression**: Cat Stretch (2 sets of 10 repetitions), Arm Circles (2 sets of 10 repetitions each side)
5. **Cool Down**: Spine Stretch (2 sets of 8 repetitions)

Tailoring Your Practice

Tailoring your Pilates Reformer routine to your specific fitness goals involves understanding your needs, selecting the right exercises, and continuously adapting your practice. By focusing on flexibility, strength, endurance, or rehabilitation, you can achieve targeted improvements and maximize the benefits of your Reformer workouts.

Chapter 7: Common Challenges and Solutions

Overcoming Plateaus

Tips for Breaking Through Fitness Plateaus

Hitting a plateau can be one of the most frustrating aspects of any fitness journey, including Pilates. A plateau occurs when you stop seeing progress despite maintaining your regular workout routine. This can happen for various reasons, such as your body adapting to the exercises, lack of variety in your routine, or insufficient challenge. Here are some tips to break through these plateaus and continue progressing:

1. **Introduce Variety**: Changing your routine can shock your muscles and encourage growth. Try incorporating new exercises, different workout sequences, or varying your workout intensity.
2. **Increase Resistance**: Gradually increase the resistance on your Pilates Reformer to challenge your muscles and promote strength gains.
3. **Focus on Form**: Sometimes, a plateau can be due to improper form. Ensure you are performing each exercise with precision and control to maximize effectiveness.
4. **Add Intensity**: Incorporate higher-intensity exercises or increase the pace of your workouts. Interval training can also help in overcoming plateaus.
5. **Set New Goals**: Establishing new, more challenging goals can motivate you to push harder and break through the stagnation.

6. **Rest and Recover**: Ensure you are getting adequate rest between workouts. Overtraining can lead to plateaus, so allow your body time to recover.
7. **Monitor Nutrition**: Proper nutrition plays a crucial role in your performance and recovery. Ensure you are eating a balanced diet that supports your fitness goals.
8. **Seek Professional Guidance**: A Pilates instructor or personal trainer can provide new insights and personalized strategies to overcome plateaus.

By implementing these strategies, you can break through plateaus and continue to see improvements in your Pilates practice and overall fitness.

Adjustments for Injuries and Limitations

Modifications for Common Injuries and Physical Limitations

Injuries and physical limitations should not deter you from maintaining an active lifestyle. Pilates is highly adaptable, and with the right modifications, you can continue to practice safely and effectively. Here are some common injuries and limitations, along with suggested adjustments:

1. **Lower Back Pain**:
    o **Modifications**: Avoid exercises that involve excessive spinal flexion, such as the Roll-Up. Focus on strengthening the

core with gentle exercises like the Pelvic Curl and Spine Stretch.

- o **Alternative Exercises**: Perform exercises that maintain a neutral spine, such as the Footwork and Leg Circles.

2. **Knee Pain**:
   - o **Modifications**: Avoid deep knee bends and high-impact exercises. Opt for low-impact movements that strengthen the muscles around the knee.
   - o **Alternative Exercises**: Use the Jump Board with light resistance for cardio without strain. Include the Leg Press on the Reformer for controlled strengthening.

3. **Shoulder Injuries**:
   - o **Modifications**: Avoid exercises that put excessive strain on the shoulders, such as the Long Stretch and the Plank.
   - o **Alternative Exercises**: Focus on gentle arm movements and shoulder stabilization exercises, such as the Arm Circles and the Chest Expansion.

4. **Wrist Pain**:
   - o **Modifications**: Avoid exercises that require weight-bearing on the wrists, like the Plank and the Push-Up.
   - o **Alternative Exercises**: Use padded supports or modify exercises to reduce wrist pressure. Focus on strengthening the forearms and maintaining wrist mobility.

5. **Hip Pain**:

- o **Modifications**: Avoid exercises that involve excessive hip flexion or extension, such as the Teaser.
  - o **Alternative Exercises**: Perform gentle hip-opening exercises and focus on strengthening the surrounding muscles with exercises like the Bridging and the Clam.
6. **Limited Flexibility**:
   - o **Modifications**: Use props like yoga blocks and straps to assist in reaching and holding positions.
   - o **Alternative Exercises**: Gradually work on flexibility with gentle stretches and mobility exercises, such as the Hamstring Stretch and the Butterfly Stretch.

Personalized Approach

Everyone's body is different, and it's essential to listen to your own body's signals and adjust accordingly. If you experience pain or discomfort, modify the exercise or consult a Pilates instructor for personalized advice. The key is to continue moving safely and effectively, even with limitations.

Part 5: Integrating Pilates into Your Lifestyle

Chapter 8: Integrating the Reformer into Your Fitness Routine

Creating a Balanced Workout Schedule

How Often to Use the Reformer

Integrating the Pilates Reformer into your fitness routine requires thoughtful planning to ensure a balanced and effective workout schedule. The frequency and duration of your Reformer sessions depend on your fitness goals, experience level, and overall health. Here are some guidelines to help you create an optimal schedule:

1. **Beginner Level**:
   - **Frequency**: Start with 2-3 sessions per week.
   - **Duration**: Each session can be 30-45 minutes long.
   - **Focus**: Concentrate on learning the basic exercises and proper form. Allow your body time to adapt to the new movements and build foundational strength.
2. **Intermediate Level**:
   - **Frequency**: Increase to 3-4 sessions per week.
   - **Duration**: Each session can be 45-60 minutes long.
   - **Focus**: Start incorporating more challenging exercises and increasing the intensity of your workouts. Aim to improve your endurance, flexibility, and overall strength.
3. **Advanced Level**:
   - **Frequency**: Aim for 4-5 sessions per week.

- Duration: Each session can be 60-75 minutes long.
- **Focus**: Push your limits with advanced exercises and variations. Focus on maintaining precise form and integrating complex movements that challenge your coordination and control.

Balancing Pilates with Other Forms of Exercise

To achieve a well-rounded fitness routine, it's essential to balance your Reformer workouts with other types of exercise. This ensures that all aspects of your fitness are addressed, including cardiovascular health, muscular strength, flexibility, and mental well-being.

1. **Cardiovascular Exercise**:
   - **Incorporation**: Include 2-3 days of cardio exercise per week, such as running, cycling, swimming, or brisk walking.
   - **Benefits**: Cardiovascular exercise improves heart health, boosts endurance, and aids in weight management.
2. **Strength Training**:
   - **Incorporation**: Add 2-3 days of strength training per week, focusing on different muscle groups each session.
   - **Benefits**: Strength training increases muscle mass, enhances metabolic rate, and improves bone density.
3. **Flexibility and Mobility**:

- o **Incorporation**: Integrate flexibility and mobility exercises daily or at the end of your workouts. This can include yoga, dynamic stretches, and foam rolling.
  - o **Benefits**: Enhances range of motion, reduces the risk of injury, and aids in muscle recovery.
4. **Mind-Body Practices**:
  - o **Incorporation**: Include practices such as yoga or meditation 1-2 times per week.
  - o **Benefits**: Promotes relaxation, reduces stress, and improves mental clarity and focus.

Sample Weekly Workout Schedule

Here's a sample weekly workout schedule that incorporates the Pilates Reformer along with other forms of exercise:

- **Monday**:
  - o Morning: Reformer Pilates (45 minutes)
  - o Evening: Light cardio (30 minutes of brisk walking or cycling)
- **Tuesday**:
  - o Morning: Strength training (upper body focus)
  - o Evening: Flexibility exercises (20 minutes of stretching)
- **Wednesday**:
  - o Morning: Reformer Pilates (60 minutes)
  - o Evening: Yoga or meditation (30 minutes)

- **Thursday**:
  - Morning: Strength training (lower body focus)
  - Evening: Light cardio (30 minutes of swimming or jogging)
- **Friday**:
  - Morning: Reformer Pilates (45 minutes)
  - Evening: Dynamic stretching (20 minutes)
- **Saturday**:
  - Morning: Long cardio session (45-60 minutes of running, cycling, or hiking)
  - Evening: Relaxation exercises (gentle yoga or meditation)
- **Sunday**:
  - Rest day or active recovery (light activity such as walking or gentle stretching)

Customizing Your Routine

It's important to customize your workout routine based on your individual needs and goals. Listen to your body and adjust the intensity and frequency of your workouts as needed. Ensure you have adequate rest and recovery time to prevent overtraining and injury.

Tips for Customization:

- **Goal Setting**: Define clear fitness goals and tailor your routine to meet those objectives. Whether you aim to improve strength, flexibility, or overall fitness, ensure your schedule aligns with these goals.

- **Flexibility**: Be flexible with your routine. Life can be unpredictable, so allow room for adjustments. If you miss a workout, don't stress—just get back on track as soon as possible.
- **Professional Guidance**: If you're unsure about how to structure your workouts, consider seeking advice from a Pilates instructor or fitness trainer. They can provide personalized recommendations and ensure you're performing exercises correctly.

Combining Pilates Reformer with Other Forms of Exercise

Incorporating a variety of exercise modalities into your routine can enhance overall fitness, improve performance, and help prevent injury. Combining Pilates Reformer workouts with cardio, strength training, and flexibility exercises creates a well-rounded fitness program that addresses all aspects of physical health. Here's an in-depth look at how to integrate these elements effectively:

1. Cardiovascular Exercise

Purpose and Benefits: Cardiovascular exercise, or cardio, is any activity that increases your heart rate and improves the efficiency of your cardiovascular system. This includes activities like running, cycling, swimming, and brisk walking. The primary benefits of cardio include:

- Improved heart health and endurance.

- Enhanced lung capacity and respiratory function.
- Increased calorie burn and weight management.
- Boosted mood and energy levels through endorphin release.

Combining with Pilates Reformer: To create a balanced fitness routine, incorporate cardio sessions 2-4 times per week, complementing your Reformer workouts. Here's how to integrate them effectively:

- **Frequency**: Alternate between cardio and Pilates Reformer workouts to allow recovery time for each system. For example, if you practice Pilates 3 times a week, you might include cardio on alternate days.
- **Intensity**: Match the intensity of your cardio workouts to your fitness level and goals. High-intensity interval training (HIIT) can be combined with Pilates for a comprehensive fitness approach.
- **Variety**: Engage in different forms of cardio to prevent monotony and target various muscle groups. Mixing swimming, cycling, and running can provide diverse cardiovascular benefits.

Sample Integration:

- **Monday**: Reformer Pilates session (45 minutes)
- **Tuesday**: Moderate-intensity cardio (30-45 minutes of cycling)

- **Wednesday**: Reformer Pilates session (45 minutes)
- **Thursday**: High-intensity cardio (30 minutes of interval running)
- **Friday**: Reformer Pilates session (45 minutes)
- **Saturday**: Low-intensity cardio (45 minutes of brisk walking or swimming)
- **Sunday**: Rest day or gentle stretching

2. Strength Training

Purpose and Benefits: Strength training involves exercises that improve muscle strength and endurance through resistance. Common methods include using free weights, resistance bands, and weight machines. The benefits of strength training are:

- Increased muscle mass and metabolism.
- Improved bone density and joint stability.
- Enhanced functional strength for daily activities.
- Greater muscle definition and improved body composition.

Combining with Pilates Reformer: Integrate strength training into your routine to complement the core and alignment focus of Pilates Reformer exercises:

- **Frequency**: Aim for 2-3 strength training sessions per week. Space them out from your Reformer workouts to allow muscle recovery.
- **Focus Areas**: Target different muscle groups on different days to ensure balanced development.

For instance, focus on upper body strength one day and lower body strength another day.

- **Intensity and Volume**: Adjust the intensity and volume of strength training based on your fitness level. Incorporate compound exercises (e.g., squats, deadlifts) that engage multiple muscle groups.

Sample Integration:

- **Monday**: Reformer Pilates session (45 minutes)
- **Tuesday**: Strength training (upper body focus, 45 minutes)
- **Wednesday**: Reformer Pilates session (45 minutes)
- **Thursday**: Strength training (lower body focus, 45 minutes)
- **Friday**: Reformer Pilates session (45 minutes)
- **Saturday**: Strength training (full body or targeted areas, 45 minutes)
- **Sunday**: Rest day or gentle stretching

3. Flexibility Work

Purpose and Benefits: Flexibility exercises improve the range of motion in your joints and muscles, enhancing overall mobility and reducing the risk of injury. Techniques include static stretching, dynamic stretching, yoga, and foam rolling. Benefits include:

- Increased joint flexibility and muscle elasticity.
- Reduced muscle tension and improved posture.
- Enhanced recovery and decreased muscle soreness.

- Greater overall body awareness and balance.

Combining with Pilates Reformer: Pilates inherently incorporates elements of flexibility, but adding dedicated flexibility work can further enhance your results:

- **Frequency**: Incorporate flexibility exercises 3-5 times a week, either as part of your warm-up or cool-down routine or on separate days.
- **Integration**: Use flexibility exercises to complement the stretching and lengthening focus of Pilates. For instance, include yoga poses or dynamic stretches before or after Reformer workouts.
- **Variety**: Explore different flexibility practices such as yoga, static stretching, or dynamic mobility drills to target various muscle groups and improve overall flexibility.

Sample Integration:

- **Monday**: Reformer Pilates session (45 minutes) followed by 15 minutes of yoga stretches
- **Tuesday**: Cardio session (30 minutes) followed by 15 minutes of dynamic stretching
- **Wednesday**: Reformer Pilates session (45 minutes) with a focus on flexibility exercises
- **Thursday**: Strength training (upper body focus) followed by 15 minutes of foam rolling
- **Friday**: Reformer Pilates session (45 minutes) with additional yoga poses

- **Saturday**: Cardio session (45 minutes) followed by 15 minutes of static stretching
- **Sunday**: Active recovery with gentle yoga or stretching (30 minutes)

Combining Pilates Reformer with Other Forms of Exercise

Integrating Pilates Reformer workouts with other forms of exercise creates a well-rounded fitness regimen that maximizes overall health and performance. This holistic approach leverages the strengths of Pilates while complementing it with the benefits of cardiovascular exercise, strength training, and flexibility work. Here's an in-depth guide to effectively combining these exercise modalities:

1. Cardiovascular Exercise

Purpose and Benefits: Cardiovascular exercise, or cardio, encompasses activities that elevate heart rate and improve cardiovascular health. Common forms include running, cycling, swimming, and rowing. Cardio offers numerous benefits:

- **Heart Health**: Strengthens the heart muscle, improving circulation and reducing the risk of heart disease.
- **Calorie Burn**: Increases energy expenditure, which aids in weight management and fat loss.
- **Endurance**: Enhances stamina and physical endurance for daily activities and other workouts.

- **Mood Enhancement**: Boosts mood and reduces stress through endorphin release.

Integrating with Pilates Reformer: To achieve a balanced fitness routine, combine cardio with Pilates Reformer workouts in a way that complements both:

- **Frequency and Timing**: Alternate cardio and Pilates sessions to avoid overtraining. For example, you might schedule Pilates Reformer workouts on Mondays, Wednesdays, and Fridays, while engaging in cardio on Tuesdays, Thursdays, and weekends.
- **Intensity and Duration**: Match the intensity of cardio to your fitness goals. High-intensity interval training (HIIT) can be combined with Pilates for enhanced calorie burn, while moderate-intensity steady-state cardio can provide active recovery.
- **Variety**: Incorporate different cardio modalities to prevent boredom and target different muscle groups. Cycling, running, and swimming each offer unique benefits that complement Pilates' core-focused exercises.

Sample Weekly Schedule:

- **Monday**: Reformer Pilates (45 minutes)
- **Tuesday**: HIIT Cardio (30 minutes)
- **Wednesday**: Reformer Pilates (45 minutes)
- **Thursday**: Moderate-intensity Cardio (45 minutes of cycling)
- **Friday**: Reformer Pilates (45 minutes)

- **Saturday**: Low-intensity Cardio (45 minutes of brisk walking or swimming)
- **Sunday**: Rest day or light stretching

2. Strength Training

Purpose and Benefits: Strength training involves exercises designed to build muscle mass and enhance overall strength. Techniques include using free weights, resistance bands, and weight machines. The benefits include:

- **Muscle Growth**: Stimulates hypertrophy, leading to increased muscle size and strength.
- **Bone Health**: Improves bone density and reduces the risk of osteoporosis.
- **Metabolism Boost**: Elevates resting metabolic rate, aiding in weight management.
- **Functional Strength**: Enhances the ability to perform daily activities with greater ease.

Integrating with Pilates Reformer: Incorporate strength training to complement the core and alignment focus of Pilates:

- **Frequency**: Plan strength training sessions 2-3 times per week, ensuring they are spaced out from Pilates workouts to allow muscle recovery.
- **Focus Areas**: Target different muscle groups each session to achieve balanced development. For example, alternate between upper body, lower body, and core-focused strength workouts.

- **Combination**: Utilize compound exercises (e.g., squats, deadlifts) in strength training to engage multiple muscle groups, which can synergize with the Pilates Reformer's focus on core stability and alignment.

Sample Weekly Schedule:

- **Monday**: Reformer Pilates (45 minutes)
- **Tuesday**: Strength Training (upper body focus, 45 minutes)
- **Wednesday**: Reformer Pilates (45 minutes)
- **Thursday**: Strength Training (lower body focus, 45 minutes)
- **Friday**: Reformer Pilates (45 minutes)
- **Saturday**: Strength Training (full body or targeted areas, 45 minutes)
- **Sunday**: Rest day or gentle stretching

3. Flexibility Work

Purpose and Benefits: Flexibility exercises improve joint range of motion and muscle elasticity, enhancing overall mobility and reducing injury risk. This includes activities such as static stretching, dynamic stretching, yoga, and foam rolling. The benefits are:

- **Improved Range of Motion**: Enhances flexibility and reduces stiffness in muscles and joints.
- **Reduced Muscle Tension**: Alleviates muscle tightness and improves relaxation.
- **Better Posture**: Supports better alignment and body mechanics.

- **Faster Recovery**: Aids in the recovery process and decreases muscle soreness.

Integrating with Pilates Reformer: Add flexibility work to complement the stretching and lengthening aspects of Pilates:

- **Frequency**: Include flexibility exercises 3-5 times a week, either integrated into your warm-up or cool-down routines, or as separate sessions.
- **Integration**: Use flexibility routines to enhance the Pilates Reformer exercises, which often focus on core strength and alignment. For example, incorporate yoga poses or stretching exercises before or after Pilates sessions.
- **Variety**: Explore different methods of flexibility work to address various muscle groups and enhance overall mobility.

Sample Weekly Schedule:

- **Monday**: Reformer Pilates (45 minutes) followed by 15 minutes of yoga stretches
- **Tuesday**: Cardio session (30 minutes) followed by 15 minutes of dynamic stretching
- **Wednesday**: Reformer Pilates (45 minutes) with a focus on flexibility exercises
- **Thursday**: Strength Training (upper body focus) followed by 15 minutes of foam rolling
- **Friday**: Reformer Pilates (45 minutes) with additional yoga poses

- **Saturday**: Cardio session (45 minutes) followed by 15 minutes of static stretching
- **Sunday**: Active recovery with gentle yoga or stretching (30 minutes)

Chapter 9: Maintenance and Care of the Reformer

The Pilates Reformer is a significant investment in your fitness journey, and proper maintenance is essential to ensure its longevity and optimal performance. This chapter provides a comprehensive guide to maintaining your Reformer and troubleshooting common issues to keep your equipment in excellent condition.

Routine Maintenance

1. Cleaning and Upkeep for Longevity

a. Regular Cleaning: Maintaining cleanliness is crucial for the Reformer's functionality and hygiene. Dust, sweat, and dirt can accumulate on the Reformer, potentially leading to wear and tear or unpleasant odors. Here's a step-by-step guide to effective cleaning:

- **Frame and Rails:** Wipe down the frame and rails with a damp cloth and mild soap. Avoid using harsh chemicals that might damage the finish. For stubborn stains, use a gentle abrasive cleaner, but ensure it's safe for metal surfaces.
- **Upholstery:** The upholstery should be cleaned regularly to prevent buildup of sweat and oils. Use a soft cloth or sponge with a mixture of

mild soap and water. Gently scrub the surface, then wipe with a clean, damp cloth to remove soap residue. Allow the upholstery to air dry completely before using the Reformer again.

- **Ropes and Straps:** Inspect the ropes and straps for signs of fraying or wear. Clean them by wiping with a damp cloth. If they are removable, wash them according to the manufacturer's instructions. Ensure they are fully dry before reattaching.
- **Springs:** Springs should be wiped down with a cloth to remove dust and debris. Check for any signs of rust or damage. Apply a small amount of lubricating oil to the spring mechanism if it becomes noisy or stiff, but be careful not to over-lubricate.
- **Foot Bar and Handles:** Clean the foot bar and handles with a disinfectant wipe or mild cleaning solution. Pay special attention to the areas that come into direct contact with your hands and feet.

b. Lubrication and Inspection:

- **Monthly Inspection:** Conduct a monthly inspection of the Reformer to check for any loose bolts, worn parts, or other signs of wear and tear. Tighten any loose bolts and replace worn or damaged parts as necessary.
- **Lubrication:** Apply lubricant to the moving parts of the Reformer, such as the carriage wheels and springs. Use a lubricant

recommended by the manufacturer to prevent excessive wear and ensure smooth operation.

- **Bumper and Casters:** Check the bumpers and casters for any signs of damage or wear. Ensure that the bumpers are securely attached and the casters move smoothly.

Troubleshooting Common Issues

a. Fixing Minor Problems:

- **Squeaky or Stiff Movement:**
  - **Cause:** Lack of lubrication, dust accumulation, or misalignment of the carriage.
  - **Solution:** Apply lubricant to the carriage wheels and check for any obstructions. Clean the rails and ensure the carriage is aligned properly. Adjust any misaligned parts as per the manufacturer's guidelines.
- **Uneven Carriage Movement:**
  - **Cause:** Uneven wear on the rails or springs, or incorrect assembly.
  - **Solution:** Inspect the rails for debris or damage. Clean and lubricate them as needed. Check the springs for uniform tension and adjust or replace them if necessary. Ensure the carriage is correctly installed and aligned.
- **Loose Foot Bar:**
  - **Cause:** Worn or loose mounting bolts.

- Solution: Tighten the bolts securing the foot bar. If the problem persists, inspect the mounting hardware and replace any damaged parts.

b. When to Seek Professional Help:

- **Severe Mechanical Issues:**
  - If you encounter significant mechanical problems, such as broken springs, malfunctioning resistance settings, or structural damage, it's crucial to consult a professional technician. Attempting to fix these issues yourself may lead to further damage or safety risks.
- **Electrical or Complex Problems:**
  - For Reformers with electrical components or advanced mechanisms, seek professional assistance if you experience issues beyond basic maintenance. Professionals can diagnose and repair complex issues that require specialized knowledge and tools.
- **Routine Servicing:**
  - Schedule regular servicing with a certified technician to ensure the Reformer remains in peak condition. Professional servicing can address wear and tear that may not be visible during routine maintenance and can extend the life of your equipment.

Conclusion

Recap of Key Techniques and Tips

In this comprehensive guide to mastering the Pilates Reformer, we've explored a range of techniques and tips designed to enhance your practice and ensure you get the most out of your workouts. Here's a summary of the essential points covered:

- **Understanding Pilates Principles:** We delved into the core principles of Pilates—Concentration, Control, Centering, Flow, Precision, and Breathing. These principles form the foundation of an effective Pilates practice, guiding how you engage with your body and execute each movement.
- **Applying Principles to Reformer Workouts:** The integration of these principles into your Reformer workouts is crucial for achieving optimal results. We covered how to apply Concentration, Control, Centering, Flow, Precision, and Breathing specifically to Reformer exercises to maximize their effectiveness.
- **Basic and Intermediate Reformer Exercises:** From fundamental exercises to more advanced routines, we provided step-by-step instructions and technique tips to help you build a strong foundation and progress in your practice. This included how to execute exercises correctly and avoid common mistakes.

- **Specialized Reformer Workouts:** We explored targeted workouts tailored for specific goals such as flexibility, strength, and rehabilitation. We also discussed how to customize routines to meet individual fitness needs and preferences.
- **Maintenance and Care of the Reformer:** Routine maintenance, including cleaning and lubricating, and troubleshooting common issues are essential for keeping your Reformer in top condition. We provided guidelines for maintaining your equipment and knowing when to seek professional help.
- **Integrating Pilates into Your Lifestyle:** We covered how to incorporate the Reformer into your regular fitness routine, combining it with other forms of exercise, and maintaining consistency to achieve long-term benefits.

Encouragement for Continued Practice

Maintaining and advancing your Reformer practice requires dedication and persistence. Remember that progress in Pilates is not just about physical transformation but also about enhancing your overall well-being. Embrace the journey with patience and enthusiasm, and continuously challenge yourself by setting new goals and exploring advanced techniques. Consistent practice, coupled with a mindful approach, will lead to improved strength, flexibility, and balance over time. Celebrate your achievements, no matter how small, and stay motivated by recognizing the positive impact Pilates has on your life.

Final Thoughts

The lifelong benefits of Pilates Reformer workouts extend far beyond the studio. By integrating Pilates into your lifestyle, you enhance your physical health, mental clarity, and overall quality of life. As you continue your practice, embrace the opportunity for ongoing learning and self-improvement. Pilates is a journey of discovery, not just of the body but also of the mind and spirit. Keep exploring, stay curious, and enjoy the transformative power of Pilates.

Appendices

Appendix A: Glossary of Terms

This appendix provides definitions for common Pilates and Reformer terminology, offering clarity and understanding for practitioners at all levels. Key terms include:

- **Reformer:** A piece of Pilates equipment with a sliding carriage and adjustable springs, used to perform a variety of exercises that target different muscle groups.
- **Concentration:** A Pilates principle emphasizing focused attention on the body's movements and alignment during exercise.
- **Control:** A principle that involves executing each movement with deliberate precision, ensuring that exercises are performed with proper form and technique.
- **Centering:** Engaging the core muscles to maintain stability and balance throughout each exercise.
- **Flow:** Creating seamless transitions between exercises to maintain a smooth, continuous movement throughout the workout.
- **Precision:** Performing exercises with accuracy and attention to detail to ensure effectiveness and reduce the risk of injury.
- **Breathing:** Using proper breathing techniques to support movement, enhance relaxation, and optimize performance during Pilates exercises.